Five Years
and Beyond

Surviving cancer and
moving forward

Denny Grant

Five Years and Beyond
Copyright © 2016 by Denny Grant

ISBN 978-1-934333-57-0

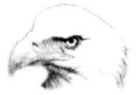

Eagle Book Bindery
Publishing Co.
Cedar Rapids, IA 52405
www.eaglebookbindery.com

This book can be purchased from
www.eaglebooks.com

DEDICATION

To my parents Bob and Immogene,

my wife Diane,

sons David and Daniel

Table of Contents

Acknowledgements

Foreword

ACKNOWLEDGEMENTS

There are so many wonderful and caring people in my life who have in one way or another inspired me to write this book. I am deeply indebted to God Almighty and my parents for giving me some humble innate abilities that enabled me to put this project together.

I especially want to thank my family and close friends and associates for their encouragement and support over the past few years. Without these caring and concerned individuals giving ideas, pointing out resources or just being there, my efforts would have likely been much more limited and the outcome far less hopeful.

I also want to acknowledge the countless number of people who are suffering or know of someone who is suffering from a protracted illness, and the hardships that they have to endure. Once you have been down this road of surprise, shock and survival, you want to give back to those who are less fortunate or those still struggling with their condition to let them know that they are not alone in their journey.

FOREWORD

Cancer, the second leading cause of death in our country, changes, damages or ends the lives of hundreds of thousands of American lives each year. Young or old, male or female, we all have been touched by someone who has this or a related disease. The new research is promising and I am very optimistic that significant breakthroughs will be made in the next 10 to 20 years that will improve the prognosis and recovery of many cancer survivors.

We are at the cusp of understanding more about the genomes of tumors and being able to suppress or eradicate their insidious efforts to ruin our lives. One of the latest developments is the use of 3D printers which can recreate a tumor likeness and therefore, treatments can be designed for it.

There is great hope in the future with the government. Vice president Joe Biden sponsored Cancer Moonshot which will be launched next year. This initiative promises to open up in a collaborative way research, medicines, clinical trials and data bases that will be geared to help those who have cancer.

This and other cutting-edge technologies can only help what was once a "death sentence" for folks who have been diagnosed with it. We are only limited by our imagination as to how to create and harness a better cancer fighting tool.

CHAPTER - I INTRODUCTION
"To thine own self be true" Shakespeare

Having been born and raised in Dubuque in the 1950s and knowing family members, ages and health histories, I never gave cancer a serious consideration as a youth. In our family we all had been fairly healthy when we were young and things like cancer and heart disease only happened to folks at an advanced age, or so I thought.

We all got the mandatory vaccinations, including the polio vaccine, but many of us still got the measles, mumps and chicken pox. We survived these conditions and had a belief system that we were in pretty good shape.

In our family there was not much talk about which grandparent or uncle had what condition. To talk about someone's health history while they were alive or even after they passed was kind of taboo. When someone died, very little was said about their legacy or health habits along the way.

It was in this climate of "mum is the word" that we were raised. We were also morally warned to not judge others, because you "never know if it can happen to you". Having a brother who was born with Down's syndrome, reemphasized this point, kind of a "don't ask don't tell" philosophy.

Our families on both sides were of northern European descent and led a fairly standard existence. We had the typical diet of the day, meat, potatoes and sometimes dessert. I also had not been exposed to any toxic agents that I was aware of. Our house was built in the 1950's and it had no known lead based paint in it.

In those days prior to hospice and palliative care, families took care of their own as an alternative of going to "a home." My paternal grandfather had died from arteriosclerosis while residing at Sunnycrest Manor in his

1

mid-seventies. My maternal grandfather, who was blind in later life and was shuttled between family members as he refused to go to a nursing home, lived to be 86.

Both of my grandparents were born in the late 19th century and had endured many hardships during their life, such as the great depression, influenza and TB outbreaks. When faced with medical issues they did not have the luxury of calling a health nurse or googling web MD. They both still lived to an advanced age, which I felt was a testament to our good family genes and luck.

It was due to my inquisitive nature that I had asked any relative that I could about the cause of death in relatives who had passed. To know health statuses, causation and age at death were just some of the things that were of interest to me during that period and which probably served me well later in my professional life in the Human service field.

My fascination with health and longevity was probably spurred on by our families' limited discussions of this topic at the supper table or other family gatherings. We had a balanced diet during those formative years and I couldn't help but wonder why some of our relatives lived longer than others. I always seemed to have an interest in how and why our kinfolk passed, especially if it seemed to be premature.

Throughout my youth and young adulthood, and up to this time, I was blessed with good health. I was able to play sports and had only one non dental surgery up until age 46. I guess that I took good health for granted and was mainly complacent about medical issues for many years. Now at the age of 62 I can only shake my head and wish that I was more aware of age related medical changes that take place as one enters middle age.

My father lived to be 79, did not take good care of his health, and had several medical conditions; but he still lived to this advanced age. I figured that he must have been blessed with good genes and luck to get that far. I, on the other hand, planned to take better care of my health and therefore live longer and hoped to be healthier.

So, with good genetics and leading a healthy lifestyle I was rolling along mostly carefree about health issues until February 1998. At that time a strange, urgent urinary sensation came over me to void. I needed to empty my bladder immediately, or face the consequences of being incontinent.

This feeling was an anomaly or so I thought. After several reoccurrences of this urinary urgency, I sought help from a local urologist. He did the usual examinations and informed me that I was diagnosed with BPH benign prostate hyperplasia and it's very common in men, especially as we age.

My urologist gave me a prescription and "voila," I felt that I was on my way to restored urinary health. I did eventually transfer to another urologist who explained how the bladder, prostate and other organs worked and what my options were. The two medications that I was prescribed during that time were designed for shrinking the prostate and relaxing the smooth muscles of the bladder.

This sounded good to me and I was cautioned to avoid caffeine and just be mindful of the BPH and risk factors associated with it. During the next 13 years, I stayed with the same urologist, and while there were some minor med changes during this time, my symptoms remained in check. The urologist reported that my prostate gland was close to normal size during the last year that I saw him.

In fall 2011, after my prostate issues seemed stable, things changed that would alter my life forever. The urologist told me that my PSA (Prostate specific antigen), which was normally .02 or less was now over 20. He saw the alarm in my face and suggested a two week script of an antibiotic because he hypothesized that this may be a false positive brought on by an infection.

We did a repeat PSA and it was higher than the prior one. The urologist expressed to me that I might have prostate cancer. It was suggested that I should have a biopsy and bone scans done to either confirm or rule out cancer.

The biopsy that was done confirmed that it was cancer. Not only was it prostate cancer but it also was spreading rapidly. The various scans confirmed this as well. The urologist had previously told me that many older guys (65+) die "with, but not from" prostate cancer and I was hoping to be in that category. We consulted several more times and he educated me on various treatment options.

He informed me that my Gleason score was (9) on a scale of 1-10. The number 10 was basically a death certificate, so now I really was scared of what may happen. I remember saying to my urologist "I need to get back to the office" as I didn't want to be late for my next appointment.

He replied, "No you don't as this cancer could take your life." This appraisal definitely got my attention and the $64,000 question was: what's our next move in dealing with this quagmire?

CHAPTER II
THE TRAUMA OF HAVING CANCER

"Always remember that you are braver than you believe and stronger that you seem and smarter than you think" Christopher Robin [1]

It goes without saying that anything that profoundly impacts a person, be it physical, emotional, psychological or spiritual, is a trauma. Dealing with the impact of cancer is more than just taking meds and seeing your doctor.

Depending on the type and location, it will affect a person at his or her deepest level. The feeling of being violated by this unwanted disease is quite profound. The very nature of one of your own cells becoming "radicalized" and multiplying and ravaging other cells, tissues, organs and ultimately taking your life is scary.

All of your good intentions as a scout, neighbor, brother, grandchild, father, mother or sibling seems to be discounted when you are dealing with various stages of this disease.

Everything is swirling around you and it's a surreal feeling when the biopsy has been completed and there is no doubt that you have cancer. Of course there are dozens of types of cancer and four main stages of progression, but nevertheless every corner of your life will be changed.

Your mind wants answers, your heart feels betrayed, your body may be in the process of being ravaged and you will be tested like never before. As a person having cancer, for the first time, you are probably thinking that there is nothing like it and nothing to compare it to.

Your faith in God or the divinity may also be called into question. This is normal during the anger stage of grief

---

[1] English author A. A. Milne has written "Winnie the Pooh" and various other poems

5

and loss. This type of thinking may permeate your thought processes for a while and coexists with your extreme terror and confusion.

Those negative or cynical thoughts will be streaming in live time, but just let them pass by. You need to stay grounded and use rational thinking during this whole ordeal. Do not let the emotional flavor of the day ruin your outlook. Stay on course with prayer, reflection, purposeful and meaningful action and a belief that all things happen for a reason.

I'm in my fifth year as a cancer survivor and it continues to astonish me as to how much a person thinks and acts differently. We see the world with new filters and guarded optimism. Hope is often mitigated with pain, fatigue and a longing for a remission. We want to get beyond this ordeal as soon as we can.

The initial diagnosis of cancer is a little like the terror attacks in Europe or elsewhere, in that a peaceful community experiences an explosion at an airport, mall or concert and much mayhem and death ensues. The entity then scrambles to restore peace and security but at the same time it is in desperate search for the perpetrators. The trauma has left an indelible imprint.

The difference, of course, is that with a terrorist attack it is all external to you and there are many intelligent systems that need to come together as a unified whole to track down the bad guys and to prevent further attacks. The city and their mood has been altered and its citizens are hoping for a quick return to the serenity that they once had.

Cancer for me has been a quirky and unpredictable illness. There are many treatments on the market and many tales of full remission and restoration of a person's prior life. Everybody's cancer is different and, no matter what you brought to the table in terms of wealth, status or strength, cancer has grabbed your undivided attention and is a formidable foe.

You don't have the luxury of the whole world helping you to heal. You are often on your own to ponder your next move or to review past treatments. Setting up some of your own protocols, with time frames can be helpful.

I think for me the trauma of having cancer is like experiencing a feeling of being lost or adrift. It sometimes seems like there are long stretches between appointments with your medical providers. You may initially feel uncomfortable with all the weeks, months and years where you won't let yourself entertain any type of "doomsday" scenarios.

Like a sailor on the ocean you are looking for a sign of land or a sea gull with an olive branch. Anything that can give you hope and a feeling of security is welcome relief. The mind will register and welcome it before the body acknowledges it.

Sometimes motivation is difficult, especially with pain and fatigue issues. You may have sleep problems and your dreams may appear to be omens of your demise. Things like advanced directives and palliative care could cross your mind, as well.

Many of us might go back to the initial biopsy and diagnosis and relive each event and word looking for answers or trying to piece together what went wrong in our lives; why we did not correct it when we should have.

All of the above situations and many more like them are completely "normal" for myself and millions of others who have been diagnosed with cancer. It's so important for all of us with cancer to gear our thought streams to positive images and focus our energy on future oriented restorative conceptions. Remember, positive imagery with specific recovery visions will serve to help you and the converse is true also.

If you find yourself stuck with any stage of grief, or emotional numbness, anger, boredom, or depressed feelings, it may be time to seek professional assistance.

Sometimes while having distressing feelings it's natural to seek comfort through food, medicine, alcohol or drugs. Obviously this is not helpful in the long run but is often understandable when we are developing sets of coping skills to offset a formidable foe.

Mental health professionals can offer private and confidential services and can be an invaluable support to help you through your "dark times." They can facilitate your own development of supports and validate your feelings and experiences, among other things.

There is no shame in asking for help. Your oncologist or primary care physician might be very good but their time and expertise may be limited for psychological based issues. Looking around for a therapist who will do an assessment and work with you to determine what could be the best course of treatment for you may be a smart idea.

It's also possible that you could need an assessment by a psychologist and/or psychiatrist to help address your emotional and mental health needs. There are also support groups in our community and nationwide that can be a safe starting point for many people. Finding a group that is a good fit for you is a big plus in so many ways.

Hearing others stories and interacting with them is like being present in a live blog but potentially a lot more rewarding, in that you are interacting with real folks. Cancer survivors giving support to others not only can have a life enhancing effect, but you can also form close fellowships.

I am continually amazed at how when we share a crisis or strong emotional experiences with others such as being pregnant or being deployed in a war zone or having cancer, can forge lasting bonds far beyond the normal neighborly or workplace connections.

CHAPTER III
STAYING ON THE GRID
"When you come to a fork in the road take it."
Yogi Berra[2]

After having been diagnosed with BPH and taking medication on a daily basis and seeing my local urologist 1 to 2 times per year for several years, I assumed that life would be good again and "this too shall pass."

I was still feeling good otherwise and being in my late 40s, these types of anomalies seemed normal to me. During the next several years my urinary issues (and my extensive prostate issues) had settled down.

I was doing exactly as the urologist had suggested and believed strongly that my prognosis for defeating this condition and avoiding other related conditions was very good. Voiding for me was reverting back to how it was prior to 1998 and that was very reassuring. I felt pretty good that the urinary problems that I had experienced were well managed and decided to let it go at that.

The types of medicines prescribed for me and others who have similar conditions were of two basic varieties: Muscle relaxers for the smooth muscles of the urinary tract area and medicine designed to shrink the prostate gland.

It was back to "business as usual" and for me during those years of having prostate and urinary issues. I did little to no research and asked few questions. I figured the condition was contained and I could focus on other priorities.

Looking back, I probably subconsciously did not want to know what other urinary and prostate issues could statistically await someone with my condition. During those first years after being diagnosed, working, raising a family,

---

[2] Yogi Berra is a Hall of fame baseball player known for his humorous sayings.

playing golf and living the "good life" was all that mattered, or so I thought.

I always kept in mind that no other immediate family members had any types of cancer that I knew of, so why worry? It felt easy to get complacent and just not stress about the unknown. In retrospect it would be prudent to continuously research and question the treatment and disease progression options.

I have since come to believe that you can never know enough about your health, and self-educating along the way can pay off in later years. Also, paying closer attention to toxins in the environment and dietary considerations must be on your check list to anyone going down this path.

"Forewarned is forearmed" as the old saying goes and I find it wise to read labels, do research and to be a critical thinker. Also challenging medical providers and getting second opinions for major things is smart.

Moving within the treatment grids, different providers and managed care companies policies and philosophies initially was frustrating to me. Why, I thought, would illnesses so important, be dealt with so casually by MCO's and in a businesslike manner by providers? I very much still felt blessed in my life and was hopeful for a positive outcome, but was increasingly wary of who was providing what kind of care and to what end. At some point I decided to just stay positive and grateful for what I had, what was available to me and others with similar conditions and not sweat the unknown. Denial can be a good, but temporary, coping skill.

Doing a systems review was the next step for me. Sizing up who can do what, and with what expertise they possess, was critically important. In Dubuque, word of mouth goes a long ways, and all of us have varying opinions of our providers and anecdotes to back up recommendations.

It's really important to not get discouraged, document well, build coalitions with the network that you are in and learn to read and research what is going on with you so you can ask legitimate questions of your providers.

Remembering that there is no such thing as a dumb question and it's always good to be polite and respectful to whomever you encounter in the medical establishments that you visit, are good adages to live by. Being assertive but not outspoken may help you to maximize your outcomes with insurance personnel that you deal with.

Many of us are almost stupefied when we are seeking our physician and are reluctant to ask tough questions or request a second opinion. We might feel that we are not worthy of help or that the medical professional have more important concerns.

We might even feel a little intimidated by them or want them to approve of us and these thoughts should give way to a more mature perspective that medical providers work for you and are duty bound to provide the best medical care, regardless of your financial situation or social status.

I have found it helpful to create a diagram of PSAS and medicine, surgical, radiographic scans and other developments that a person has endured over the years. This big picture view is beneficial for your own information as well as seeing the scope of services performed.

Sharing this diagram with your oncologist can help the both of you see the direction and progress of your illness and the treatments that have been provided to you. With the advent of online charts, the patient can access much information in cyberspace and this too can be very helpful.

Doing a semi-annual or yearly review of your medical conditions and reflecting on your progress is smart. Keep in mind that your illness does not define you, no more than a pro athlete is defined by his or her statistical prowess.

I often like to reflect as to the who, what, where, when and why. The last question is the toughest and that is where having faith and spirituality may be the healing balm to help a person through dark times of his or her disease state.

Your energy, focus and attention is best served working with what you have (not what you want) and being mindful of what you can and cannot control. It's amazing the amount of open-minded referrals to non-network providers that many insurance companies will allow. If you don't ask, they will not offer, but like Dorothy and her three friends in the Wizard of Oz, often your wishes can be granted.

It also never hurts to inquire and appeal, if you believe that going to different providers to get second opinions is what you need. Being sincere on the phone and having your facts in order could facilitate getting insurance companies to grant your request. Paying bills on time and being respectful to your MCO staff can pay off for you as well. You may need to plead your case in some circumstances.

Being mindful of your medical benchmarks is also important to be aware of. Many of us get routine lab and blood work, bone scans, MRIs and other assessments as needed that are worked into our treatment regime by our physicians and insurance companies as part their best practice protocol. The key issue is getting the most effective intervention at the proper time to ensure your safety and in keeping with your medical treatment needs.

You have to be cognizant of what you want from your treatment in terms of outcomes and symptom reduction and how your insurance company can best assist you with your stated goals. Taking full ownership of your medical options and utilizing them to the fullest should be one of your "bucket list" agenda items. Compiling the risks/benefits of each intervention can also be helpful.

Along the way you might have heard vignettes of others with similar conditions and what their medical provider prescribed for them or people with very good health care plans and what treatment options they were able to access.

A caveat here is that not everyone has the same options and we are all different folks and need to try to not get stressed out with a "grass is greener" attitude. Just do the best you can with what you've got and be happy with that!

CHAPTER IV
DEALING WITH EMOTIONS
"Sweet Emotion" Aerosmith[3]

When you are in the healing profession for a few decades you become trained to compartmentalize and utilize "detached concern." This practice allows most of what you deal with from others to be filtered to your unconscious vault, and can be dredged up if need be.

There are sometimes breakthrough situations, but you know early on if you are taking too much of your job home and, if that is the case, then perhaps you should consider another profession.

It's when the crisis strikes home, and it's your "bacon" on the bubble when things get real in a hurry. There is a lot to be said about what a person goes through when it's you who has a potentially life threatening illness. Theory gives way to reality and action is needed.

We are all familiar with the grief and loss process as defined by many different authors. The first stage is shock and denial followed by bargaining, anger, depression and ultimately acceptance. These stages can be reversed by situational triggers.

Depending on the type of cancer, medical history, age and gender of the person, many different reactions will take place. To be sure there is a torrent of emotions and a sense of being in the Twilight Zone, but there is no one to say "picture a man who thought he was going to die but woke up to a bad dream."

Having the energy to continue your quest is just one of the many assets that you may need going forward. Having faith that things will be as they are going to be and that your

---

[3] Aerosmith is a world famous musical group

destiny is already been pre-determined is a philosophical angle that has merit, in my opinion, and might help to alleviate the angst of the thoughts that you have total control over your destiny.

Remember, there is no tool bar or decision tree to precisely decide what is best for you. Somewhere in the intersection of medical, spiritual, family, research and educated guesses is where you will probably make most of your decisions.

Letting your emotions rule you or making snap choices when you are desperate, depressed or pressured may not end up as positive for you. I needed to back away and weigh the options of surgery, radiation or nothing at all and I was not given much time to make that choice.

With a Gleason score of 9 and given the diagnosis of Stage 4 cancer, there was a sense of urgency. My emotional mind ruled for a bit but eventually I believe that discussing my situation with family, colleagues and friends gave me quick pause to reflect and the wise choice was made.

There will be folks who get cancer and who see this diagnosis as a relief and an opportunity to exit an unhappy life. For some poor souls who have long since wanted to have their emotional or physical pain end, they can look forward to getting their wish. After their diagnosis is made, their life's defining moment will be an escape to the hereafter, whatever that might be.

The best most of us can do is contain and try to understand our feelings and temper these within the dichotomy of living or dying. We often feel utterly dependent upon medical providers to give us treatment, guidance, direction and some degree of hope. Their words of wisdom or experience can make or break our day.

Emotions could come in waves of blank intensity or alternate between sadness, hopelessness, powerlessness, anger, fear, fleeting optimism etc. Sometimes a person will get stuck with one or another of these negative feelings or be in a spiral of pessimistic clusters of emotions.

People may perceive their condition totally beyond their control and replace a sense of mastery with cynicism and sarcasm instead of being optimistic and confident. To my way of thinking, there is always hope for either a cure or remission or symptom relief, but I also have been down that "dark path" to the black hole of hopelessness and it's not fun.

If a person does "bottom out" with his or her emotions so that hopelessness and powerlessness are the most prevalent feelings, it's time to seek help or take drastic measures to get well and stable again. To feel disaffected by this illness can be stressful much of the time.

For most of us being aware of the triad of body, mind and spirit can be useful. Remembering that all three of these domains can act independently or in concert with the other two may provide positive or negative synergy for you.

If you are struggling with your faith, health, or spirit, the other spheres of your being will most certainly be adversely affected. In all likelihood, you would want the guidance of a professional counselor or member of the clergy to help you get to your healing "sweet spot."

This is a place where and when all of the positive energies of your three domains coalesce to lift you as a person to a more healthy place. I believe that it takes a lot of thought and concerted effort to create the optimal circumstances that are most conducive to your body's healing system to get this fully functioning state activated. For most of us, it's a fluid and ongoing process that never ends, but we can sense by our intuition that our general well-being is improving and our prognosis is on the upswing.

CHAPTER V
EFFECTS ON SPOUSES AND FRIENDS
"All I Need is a Miracle"
Mike and the Mechanics[4]

After the cancer diagnosis is made and you begin the tedious process of informing important persons in your life of your situation, it reality hits home that this is "not a drill." Your spouse and family will hopefully show caring and concern and be a buffer with the bad news and a cheerleader for the good.

The parallels with grief and loss are definitely there. There are stages and milestones that all of us with chronic debilitating illnesses go through. A surreal aura may surround a person for a while that this must be a dream.

Sometimes people will ask right away "How are you doing?" A brief update on your progress, medicine and scans are in order. Generally I have found that when family and well-meaning friends are checking for an update they are looking for some encouraging sign or disease change to boost your spirits.

Any positive anecdote that you can share will provide relief for you and your support. The takeaway from these interactions is that folks are well intentioned and you should be inclined to respond to their positive inquiries with grace. They often hold views that might reinforce or enhance yours.

The effects on your significant other is similar and different from the impact on family and friends. In my case, having been married over 25 years and having grown kids out of the house, was probably an easier scenario than if we were young parents. I did not have to immediately worry

---

[4] Mike and the Mechanics is a rock and roll band based in the U.K.

about kids in school, who need both parents for so many of life's challenges.

Forging a close collaborative bond with your significant other is good strategy for the both of you. Trusted confidants are there for your support, encouragement and as a hedge against your feeling sorry for yourself or wallowing in the "what ifs."

There are many important discussions that need to take place with your partner. There's your diagnosis and prognosis, advanced directives, will and testament among other things.

It's imperative to be inclusive and prepare for the worst-case scenario but plan, pray and hope for the opposite. Telling your significant other what you need from him or her is important for the progress updates and so that you both can move forward.

Reviewing your insurance policies (health, life and home) in a businesslike way will be empowering for you, the spouse and your survivors. Having the luxury to make informed choices now is a great vehicle to determine vital options, for when "that time" comes.

Laying out all of your emotional and financial cards on the table is a win/win proposition. The best decisions are made here. You get to check off what you want and don't want and how you want this accomplished. Just think of the chaos if you would die suddenly and there was not 100% clarity with your survivors.

It goes without saying that your disease affects the whole family. They are with you in thought and prayer, and for this you must be grateful. You and your family will likely be having discussions about life and death. Incorporating these into family traditions and legacy issues is also very important.

You may want to review your family tree and have conversations with your family members about your genealogy. This is partly an update for now, but in the future could be helpful to your heirs. They have a socio-familial need to know your medical history, especially when they gather to "celebrate your life."

Your traditional role within your family and social network is also evolving with the progression of your cancer or disease state. Whereas once you may have been the mover and shaker, now you head to the lazy boy and you might have tremors from the medicine.

Adjusting to and accepting these changes has been the biggest challenge for me and others with similar conditions. Understanding that what has transpired was no one's fault. Having to give up your career and retirement preferred choices is also part of the balance sheet change in your life.

Overall, I considered myself to have been fortunate and blessed during the past several decades. Continuing that train of thought and expanding it to more spiritual and gratitude oriented reflections has been a growth process for me.

Gone are the days of playing 36 holes of golf or jogging down the street with little effort. Now more and more my days are filled with quiet, family and home activities that involve conversation and light exertions. This is becoming more acceptable as time goes on.

Remember you deserve this retirement time to pause, reflect, and be open to healing and accepting a "new normal." You are still you but you may have a new persona and outlook.

Another of the important paradoxical lessons that I have learned from my ordeal is to be thinking in terms of the "gifts of cancer." While this may seem to be ironic at first blush there are undoubtedly some positive things that can come from having cancer or other debilitating illnesses.

This is not to suggest that we want to contract M.S., diabetes, Crohn's disease or other unpleasant afflictions. If however a person gets an illness where they have to negotiate employment, familial and social realities, and they have time on their hands, there is room for spiritual growth.

Viewing your illness from a rational lens is normal and quite expected. Acquiring a condition in which you are traumatized and your life is turned upside down is a very difficult proposition to feel positive about.

There could come a time in your healing journey in which you or the significant other come to see the condition as a challenge but also an opportunity. From a spiritual perspective there may be new horizons of purpose and meaning to be extracted. Having an open mind to defocus on medical issues and refocus on spiritual things can be a "game changer" that keeps you sane.

The past 4 1/2 years have yielded an unexpected harvest of new purpose and meaningful endeavors for me. This epiphany did not happen overnight. After going through the grief and loss stages, and "what now" rhetorical questions I have come to the belief that things do happen for a reason and we can find goodness and value in almost anything.

I try hard to no longer be troubled with transient or small issues. Remembering that all stuff is "small stuff" can be helpful. For many of us in this hectic world of deadlines and productivity pressures, getting deprogrammed is not only useful but almost essential if you have a life-threatening illness and want to live your future in a useful and purposeful way.

The most important things to you may be your spiritual life, family and friends. Money and material things come and go. Your sports team might lose a close game, the neighbors may be loud on occasion and the politician you least like, may have been elected.

The human part of us might react and experience some emotions over the circumstances listed above. We should reorient ourselves to a new belief mindset that happiness, success and contentment are important to our human existence, but not to our spiritual existence.

CHAPTER VI
DUAL CRISIS
"Monday, Monday"
The Mommas and Papas[5]

They say when it rains it pours and bad things come in three's. I'm just glad that only the first cliché was applicable here. For me the co-occurring crisis besides my cancer was my mother's rapidity deteriorating health. She was 92 years old and was residing in a local nursing home for the past two years.

She had been diagnosed with Alzheimer's disease years before and had resided in a residential living facility next to an ICF facility. Moving there was a relatively smooth transition for her, but tough for her family and one big step towards her inevitable passing.

Being a doting son for a wonderful role model and parent, it was a no brainer visiting her on Sundays. These were wonderful bonding times and opportunities to give back all the love and caring that she so willingly shared with us growing up.

There were six boys and we all felt blessed that she ensured our educational, social and spiritual involvement whilst we were growing up. She never had a bad thing to say to others and went to church daily if possible.

My mother's declining health in late 2011 coincided almost exactly with my cancer diagnosis and subsequent deterioration. It was a scramble for myself to continue to work on a full-time basis, pay attention to my medical needs and to maintain regular contact with my mother's nursing and hospice staff.

---

[5] Monday, Monday was sung by "The mamas and papas"

Sometime in January 2012, mom was not responsive to conversation, was not eating and was slipping away before our eyes. We had been very pleased with hospice's attention to detail for her care and our needs.

They facilitated medical and spiritual connections during her final days, and for that we were very grateful. During the same month of January 2012, I was faced with a life or death struggle with my own rapidly progressing prostate cancer.

With family and my friend Erin's suggestions for a second opinion outside of Dubuque, I was screened and approved for a relatively new procedure using "robotics" with the Da Vinci method. This cancer clinic was located in Madison, Wisconsin at the University of Wisconsin medical center.

Being that UW - Madison is a nationally certified cancer treatment center, and having had its approval for this surgery, I opted to have the prostatectomy done there. Since this facility was only 90 miles away and since I had heard good things about it, the choice seemed easy. The staff and team of physicians were friendly and very familiar with patients with my condition and status.

The date for the surgery was set for Valentine's Day 2012. My mother passed away on January 30, 2012 just 15 days prior to my surgery. We had her funeral on my older brother Rod's birthday, as it just worked out that way.

The funeral mass, wake service and funeral were very dignified and I believe conducted with the highest level of reverence and respect due her. It was a relief that I no longer had to worry about her health concerns.

I comforted myself with thoughts of delaying doing the proper grief work for her after my surgery and recovery, so as to be able to devote every measure of thoughts and emotions where they were needed most urgently.

CHAPTER VII
D DAY OF SURGERY
"Are You Man Enough" Four Tops[6]

The day of the surgery approached rapidly and, even though I was dreading it, there was no doubt that if I did not have this surgery, I would likely die. My wife, Diane rode with me to the campus at UW Madison on a cold Valentine's Day. We checked in and spoke with the administration and medical staff.

I was put in a private exam room and administered an IV by a nurse who eventually also hooked up to anther IV containing a sedative, and this got me relaxed in a hurry. Shortly thereafter, medical staff pushed my wheeled bed rapidly to the OR, and as I observed many lights inside it and within five seconds, I was unconscious.

I awoke after about two hours in a recovery room with a catheter in me while sitting up in a hospital bed. Diane was there to keep me company and that was a welcome sight. The hospital also allowed her to stay the night on a rollout bed in my room.

Staff were friendly and attentive to my needs. It was actually nice ordering off the menu and getting ice cream and other treats. I did have a sense of "enjoy this while it lasts" as I knew the hard work was yet to come.

During my surgery my older brother Rod had driven up from Dubuque and we visited in my room. It was very comforting to see him, as he is a great source of support. Another brother Paul, who lives in Texas had sent flowers to my room to cheer me up. It was heartwarming to have those, as well.

---

[6] Are You Man Enough sung by the group Four Tops

Many medical staff had come in to check my progress and status and to keep me informed as to what to expect. Overall the staff were professional and caring.

The fun was over the next day as I was wheeled out of my room to be discharged. It was Diane, myself and the catheter getting into my car. This painful device was a sore reminder of what I had just endured and among the five incision sites, two were "weeping" and these were not tears of joy. The pus was oozing out of these sites for more than a week and it was also very uncomfortable.

I was very worried about getting an infection and did my best to keep the surgery sites clean. I also needed to change and clean the catheter several times per day and this was also very stressful but necessary. The pain of the catheter was exceeded by the worry of infection and the oozing.

As part of the discharge plans the hospital staff had previously told me to eat something and be active and exercise when I returned home. They also indicated that typically after surgery the bowels need to "wake up" before they function at their best. It was a struggle to get all of the "plumbing" working for the next nine days.

At that time I returned to the UW as a post op follow-up and also to get the dreaded catheter removed. Staff completed this and at my request, the surgeon wrote a letter to my urologist stating that "external low beam radiation" was no longer indicated and that using a variety of anti-cancer medicines was the recommended treatment route going forward.

This recommendation applied in 2012. But in 2016, faced with metastasizing cancer again this time in the "pubic bone" radiation was now the treatment of choice. I said my final hospital farewells, and expressed appreciation to al] that the staff at UW did. I knew that there was a lot of recovery work ahead.

I was told by the Dubuque and UW staff that if one cancer cell "escaped" the surgery it could migrate and multiply and metastasize. Even though I no longer had a prostate gland. I could theoretically have a relapse of prostate cancer somewhere else in my body.

The time spent in the hospital was time to reflect mentally and spiritually while my body was healing physically. One might tend to over analyze these types of situations and dwell on problem-solving strategies or coping mechanisms.

Looking back, probably the time best spent for me would just be relaxing and enjoying each moment in a "mindfulness" framework. I had to remind myself that this is a journey and there will be many stops along the way and there are not always answers or solutions readily available.

Finding that inner peace and safe place would be the best suggestion for this part of the post-surgery progress, as far as I am concerned. Remembering all the love, kindness and goodness, and allowing those warm feelings to restore an optimistic outlook is also time well spent. Too often in the rush and chaos of everyday, we can take for granted the many blessings that most of us have in our life.

Securing and nurturing that safe place and inner peace that often comes with healing, especially after surgery, is also time well used. If nothing else, I learned that having gratitude and developing myself spiritually would be some of the best things to do.

There are things in this life we can control but the ones that we can't are the scariest. Not having choices that are difference makers was tough for me to come to terms with. Looking back daily moments of gratitude and prayer helped to dissipate the bad thoughts.

CHAPTER VIII
HEALING AND RECOVERY POST-OP
"I've Seen Fire and I've Seen Rain"
James Taylor[7]

After I had been released from the hospital, it was time for the real healing to begin. The hospital and doctors gave me written instructions to follow post -op and resource numbers to call. They offered suggestions to ease my discomfort and to promote healing.

It was very important for me to follow these directions and to be my own best advocate. Having had prostate and cancer issues like I had, terms like pain management, PSA'S, bone scans become important terms going forward.

As a patient you, your urologist and oncologist team will have to have an understanding as to what the radiographic numbers mean and when more invasive or aggressive treatments are indicated. There will be protocols customized for you and most medical treatment teams are well established. But it would be a mistake to put your total faith in your practitioners. Trust but verify with your own research.

Sometimes mistakes are made and, although many great providers are out there, you have to establish the "what" and the "who" and how they work for you. You are not financially obligated to stay with a nurse, clinic or physician and getting second opinions is now the norm. Ask tough questions and continue to seek the best providers available. You deserve it and there are usually no "do overs."

---

[7] "Fire and Rain" sung by James Taylor

At this point, because your life will be a mix of surreal moments, surrounded by fogginess and fear, you must trust that there are better days ahead. It goes without saying that having a support network of family, friends and people who know and care what you are going through and what you may be experiencing, is an invaluable source of comfort and understanding.

Even so, there will be lots of moments of feeling alone, scared and disconnected. Reminding yourself that you are still the same basic person with hobbies, interests, involvements and goals should help to keep you on the correct path.

Giving yourself reassurance that there is a higher power in play and that your recovery path will be helped by your own faith-based efforts, may also be of value to you.

Having a sense that your creator won't abandon you and believing strongly in a higher purpose, could help keep you from losing your faith based hope pathway. Even on your worst days, try not to feel like a victim or blame God for your circumstances.

Believing that there is a higher power working with each of us, helping your efforts, has helped me a great deal. Whether or not you have some type of faith, there is no denying that praying for yourself or someone else is a useful and fruitful option.

Any number of studies have shown that prayer can and has enhanced healing and often will give the person a lot of spiritual comfort. There are patron saints for cancer and passages in the Bible that you may decide to be a good fit for you.

Having left the surgical floor and having re-entered my life, there were challenges ahead for me. I was encouraged by medical and anecdotal evidence of remarkable stories of healing to the point of restoring life as it once was.

I believed ahead of time that there would be gains and losses in my recovery efforts, and I was surprised to learn how much untapped strength that each of us have. Surviving cancer and restoring as much of your prior life are noble and achievable goals. Acquiring the necessary tools and keeping a positive outlook are more doable than they would seem.

Remember these types of illness are not for weak of heart and post-op is the time to tap into the innate primal survival mechanism. It's in there, one just has to want it bad enough.

Since cancer seems for most of us to be an enigma, wrapped in a riddle surrounded by mystery, your recovery course will likely not be linear. My own healing journey is ongoing and probably anything but typical. I have found it useful to learn all I can about this condition and to embark on a course of health and wellness, no matter where that may take me. It's funny how serendipity may be in play without a person realizing it.

Even with the best supports and medical teams behind me, there are many days and weeks where there appears to be no progress or even a regression of symptoms. It's important to take one day at a time and to look at the big picture and to measure progress where you can with consistent tools.

There is no quit in cancer and, like a football game, the final outcome is often uncertain until the last play. Remember "it's not over until it's over" and many times it seems that forces beyond our control determine our destiny.

There is always hope, until you breathe your last. The stories of exceptional healing and recovery with the grimmest of prognosis, has helped to inspire me to not give up the fight. As part of my healing mandate I plan to continue to share what I have learned in my journey to help others with theirs.

CHAPTER IX
WHAT'S IN YOUR TOOL KIT?
"Rub It In, Rub It In" Billy "Crash" Craddock [8]

We all have had life experiences with success and failures. These learning episodes may serve us well in this next phase of our healing and recovery journey.

I am listing some useful skills and tools that have worked for myself and others over the years. This is by no means a complete listing of action steps or philosophies to embrace but is meant to give the reader an index of sorts as to what could be helpful for you.

If you are struggling with what to think about and how to sustain your efforts, it may be helpful to seek a therapist familiar with chronic illnesses. There are also local or national chapters dedicated to the conditions that you are currently experiencing.

Remember you are not alone In your struggle, unless you choose to be, and that would be most unfortunate. It's so much better to get the love and comfort from others and many times others have suggestions that can help immensely.

You are unique and ultimately have the final say in what you think and do. It behooves all of us with diseases to start with a foundation of basic self-care and interpersonal and life skills that are tailored to meet our needs, and are within the framework of what you have to work with.

Not everyone can be like Dr. Norman Cousins who wrote the book "Anatomy of an Illness"[9] and who survived what should have been a terminal illness.

The reader may recall that he locked himself into hotels with tapes of comedic performances that helped to ignite his immune system, enabling him to live a long life.

---

[8] "Rub it In" sung by Billy "Crash" Craddock
[9] "Anatomy of an Illness" written by Dr. Norman Cousins

Much longer than he would have had he succumbed to his illness without the lifestyle changes.

Doing a self-appraisal of your current functioning level is part of your overall assessment of what kinds of tools and lifestyle altering efforts that you need to make.

This next section of tools and ideas was written in no specific order. They are a random cross section of thoughts and concepts that I have used in my struggle with cancer over the past 4 1/2 years.

Starting with arguably the most important of these ideas is to find the best providers in your area. Practitioners or providers who have a proven track record of working with patients who have the same condition that you have is a must. Not only should these oncologists, urologists, or internal med physicians be skilled and experienced, they should also take a personal interest in you and your concerns.

If you don't believe that these doctors give a hoot about you or are just going through the motions, by all means seek a second opinion. There is usually transportation that can be arranged to more regional hospitals and clinics, if you want or need a second opinion.

Your physician who is working for and paid by you should have no problem writing a referral that may benefit you, if he or she truly cares about what's in your best interest.

It usually is smart to start with more urgent medical concerns and proceed to less urgent ones. Remember the acronym ODDD, as it will be one of the many signposts to refer to along your healing journey.

*The O refers to your organs and keeping them healthy and functioning well. Your liver, lungs, kidneys, brain and stomach all play vital roles in your body's ability to heal itself. They will keep your momentum going in the right direction and, like a durable engine, will bolster your efforts when needed.

31

*The first D relates to Documentation, especially in the doctor's office. Ask good questions and make notes of what is said, recommended or concluded. If there is a referral for lab or a bone scan, be sure to note that.

*The second D is finding a Doctor who only or primarily specializes in your condition. For years before my cancer diagnosis and for almost three years afterwards, I primarily used a urologist. He ultimately referred me to a oncologist who not only specialized in cancer issues but could give me the medicine shots that I need for my cancer.

Like a lot of folks, I liked my urologist and thought that he had all the answers. But it's important to remind yourself that friendliness is great, but where does the expertise lie?

*The last D in our acronym is Diet and specifically a modified Mediterranean is recommended by many. This is the one that is loaded with fruits, vegies, olives, legumes, and whole grains. The French fries, and Big Macs should be rare here for many reasons.

Also plenty of water and avoiding sodas and too much acid is a good idea. It's smart to check the internet and confer with your physician to double check any recommendations. Some folks are going organic and avoiding GMO'S and this sounds prudent as well. Factoring in a person's age and gender for specific nutrition is additionally recommended.

Food is your friend and food is medicine. It can work in this regard for you. Many types of berries and herbs are thought to have healing or curative properties to them and, of course besides being antioxidant many of them taste good as well.

To summarize, if you have a great diet and like it and it works for you, great, but it doesn't hurt to seek additional expertise to get that extra cancer fighting edge. I have found

Dr. Weil's[10] books very good for general health, healing and dietary suggestions.

The mind also plays a critical role in your cancer or other serious illness recovery. It's been my experience that we often get what we expect and those who are most determined often end up with what seek. Much of our expectations and outcomes are driven by ourselves.

Hard as it is to conceive, one of the first big junctions in the road for my dealing with cancer, was accepting it. This took place prior to understanding the genesis of how cancer works. Being in denial, and getting defensive about the diagnosis, took what energy and momentum that I had and it just spun me around.

I did not have much treatment traction until I realized that the cancer was not going away and this recovery would be a long one. Only then could I formulate a strategy. I had hoped that the prostatectomy surgery that was performed in Madison would cure my cancer once and for all. It took hard work to accept, understand, and channel my energies toward coping and overcoming this illness.

Cancer is more likely to beat you if you think it will. My friend, Jaro, loaned me a book written by doctors Simonton and Dr. Creighton entitled "Getting Well Again"[11]. This is a must read if you have cancer or another serious illness and you want to get well again. It outlines key strategies that are necessary for your recovery.

The use of imagery is one of the most important tools that you can use. Drawing an image of your cancer on paper and then another one in a few months can tell a lot about your view of your cancer and your recovery prospects. You are limitless as to how you can visualize cancer in abstract forms which can translate to everyday events. For example: Think of your cancer cells as lint on the floor to be sucked up by your mental image of a vacuum cleaner.

---

[10] Dr. Andrew Weil has written several books on health

[11] "Getting Well Again" by Dr.'s Simonton and Creighton

You are only restricted by your imagination as to how to think of your condition and strategies in your mind's eye. By visualizing what you perceive the nature and threat of your cancer or illness to, imagery can help direct your healing energies.

Doing imagery and using relaxation exercises can have many benefits besides tools to fight cancer. They can help lower your stress and blood pressure and therefore promote more healing. The more you awfulize about what may happen the more you won't get well.

Remember to use your "wise" mind. In theory we have emotional rational and wise minds. When we get triggered by something internal or external, we will automatically be flooded with chemicals and emotions, many of which are not conducive to getting well.

Utilizing rational thinking of feelings and events is good and necessary. Since the wise mind is at the intersection of the emotional and rational minds, going there can give us wisdom and the energy upon which to proceed towards improved health.

Trusting and treating your gut well is very important also. From my research, everyone from Hippocrates to current day physicians and nutritionists, especially those involved in holistic health are strong advocates of having a healthy gut.

Imbibing too many acidic foods and drinks will most certainly cause you discomfort in the short run and a whole array of unwanted symptoms in the long run. Foods like probiotics can help to keep a healthy balance of bacteria in the gut, where it should be.

Remember that much of your body's production of serotonin (an important neuro-transmitter for mood) is located in your gut. Also, since many of your immune system functions stem from your gut as well, it only makes sense to keep this area supplied with the nutritional items that it craves the most.

Many conditions such as IBS, colitis and indigestion are thought to originate with negative emotions, which can manifest in your gut. If you take care of your emotional and sustenance needs, your gut will likely take care of you.

Be in touch with negative emotions like anger, hatred, and chronic negativity. Try to turn these into something positive. Getting to the root causes of why you may think or feel so negative or hostile can be a turning point to your overall health. Remember the mind/body/spirit triad when reviewing your health and seek to maintain balance and healthy actions in these areas.

Regarding those negative emotions, it's important to learn how to manage them and to not let them manage you. All of what you experience emotionally is "normal" or within the usual spectrum of human interaction with or without having cancer or another serious illness.

The point that I am stressing is that establishing a pattern of negative, angry or sad feelings and thoughts is not "normal" and will be debilitating. Even if you feel justified, these toxic emotions will disrupt your social, physical and intellectual functioning.

First be aware of these negative emotions and second, find effective ways to defuse or redirect them. This is a high cognitive process that is critical for your healing responses. Talking to a counselor, pastor or other professional can be helpful in self-understanding and in the effective use of coping skills.

For many of us doing daily reflections and use of prayer, exercise, social and community activities can be helpful. Being mindful of your breathing, thoughts and urges and not allowing yourself to dwell on the past is also productive.

You can only control you and no one else. The use of prayer, forgiveness and positivity are great tools to use daily. Mastery of these concepts takes time, and in no time others will recognize the new you and your newly created persona.

Some of the aforementioned patterns that we all have can be categorized somewhat with the terms schemas, or filters. These mostly unconscious mechanisms are rooted in our past experiences and are often beyond our awareness.

These filters are listed in no particular order and we all are subject to them. You can probably Google a "do -it - yourself" filter sheet online. The main filters that we all employ are as follows: Mistrust, failure to achieve, undesirability, abandonment, unrelenting standards, subjugation, self-sacrifice, entitlement, vulnerability to harm and social defectiveness.

If you are looking into these filters and are concerned about your score, I would recommend that you see professional assistance to learn more about these and the subsequent work to help yourself become more mentally healthy.

Once we do an honest appraisal of the areas of trauma or damage that we "own" then we could be at the genesis of an improved sense of self. There may be events that have deeply troubled us, and by not processing and resolving them, we are at an increased risk of damaging our present interaction with others and ourselves.

The previously mentioned list is just the beginning of your quest along your psychological healing path. If you open your mind to thinking and perceiving your life in new and different ways, then it would seem reasonable that your chance of improving your physical health would be enhanced.

I like to keep my routine consistent and simple. Having a daily routine mostly filled with a mix of exercise, reading, spiritual and social interactions works for me. I have had to scale back physical activities like long walks and golfing due to the side effects of medications and from the cancer.

I try to keep a consistent theme in my head of "I'm not going to let this illness beat me". I certainly don't have all the answers but I have found a lot of useful information on the internet and in interacting with others who have similar conditions.

Believing in yourself and your essence is so important in your recovery and healing efforts. Remember, that cancer or any debilitating illness can cause people to doubt themselves and believe that they deserve what they got. It's very important to have the power of faith in yourself and be determined to beat your condition.

There were many dark days for me and I am grateful to have survived this long. Now I believe that I will beat my cancer and will come out the other side a healthier and more purposeful person.

CHAPTER X
REVVING UP YOUR
HEALING SYSTEM
"Hot Rod Lincoln" Commander Cody[12]

One of the things I have learned in the past few years has been the presence and function of our innate healing system. This invisible apparatus has been burnished in all of mankind since we started walking upright. It's not much of a stretch to believe that we are all endowed with an immune system and a vast network of systems to help us heal. These are hard wired in our species and are essential for our survival.

I am not learning more all the time on this subject and it's intriguing to believe that we have a great healing capacity that few of us have fully tapped. The vastness of possibilities of what could be utilized in our healing journey is worth the time and effort to know more about this.

It's likewise helpful to know your relatives and their health and disease history. Being a collector of genetic, dietary, spiritual social, life experience and medical information will be useful to all of us in a "pay it forward" arrangement.

We can't undo our genes but we can learn more about how the body heals and can stay well. Practitioners of "holistic" healing and medicine cite the allopathic use of antibiotics and the continued emphasis on disease suppression as examples of how many in our society struggle with poor health and early death.

In past days of the medical model and the triad of insurance companies, pharmacies and medical providers were arguably the most expedient mode of service delivery. With the patient, provider and payer triangle so well

---

[12] Commander Cody is a rock a roll band who plays in the U.S.

established, it was easy to buy into this treatment configuration.

We are now learning more about other (complimentary) types of medical models. Many of us have used nontraditional treatment choices like chiropractic care with good results and a few of us have dabbled into herbs, supplements and organic products.

It is becoming increasingly evident to me that the "traditional" medical establishment of clinics and offices are perhaps not the "be all, end all" for many of us. To be sure, most doctors are kind, well-meaning and well -educated when we interact with them.

My suggestion here is to think for yourself and question everything that is recommended for you. Research your medicines, side effects and conditions that you might have. It may seem to some that in our culture, we have a medical establishment that is primarily focused on disease and symptom suppression and not as much on health and healing.

Having a great and effective medical staff is to be applauded, but be mindful that not everyone and not every condition will respond to "modern medicine" and the current medical delivery models.

By now we have all heard of antioxidants, omega 3 fatty acids and free radicals. Few of us are chemists, and my point here is to do a very brief overview to underscore the importance of knowing the best foods to eat to protect and preserve your body and to enhance your immune response.

Antioxidants are substances that inhibit oxidation or remove potential damaging oxidizing agents. In other words antioxidants are contained in foods such as vitamins C, E and beta carotene and they help to offset negative efforts by the free radicals.

Free radicals are thought to be an atom or a molecule that have a single unpaired electron on their outer shell, which can affect neighboring molecules to become more free radicals. These marauding molecules can cause damage to cells and promote diseases like Alzheimer's, atherosclerosis, cancer, diabetes and arthritis.

This should scare most of us to heed the warning that negative outcomes could be headed our way if we don't do a better job to protect ourselves. The best foods to help in this process include broccoli, carrots, spinach, tomatoes, mushrooms, strawberries and blueberries. There are many others to be sure, but if most of us can start with an awareness of this potential process and what to do to protect ourselves, it would be a great benefit.

Many other cultures from China to the Amazon rain forest have had their share of healers, be they medicine men or shamans or voodoo practitioners. It's good to remember also that our country has been in existence since only the 18th century, and many other countries and cultures have predated us by thousands of years.

I strongly believe that anyone with a chronic debilitating medical condition should be looking globally for a cure or relief, if they are not getting the results they want. In this day of "google" and the internet, one can find an amazing amount of research results or anecdotal examples of how folks with life -threatening conditions somehow defy all the odds, survive and are doing well now.

I certainly am appreciative of all the wonderful care and treatment offered by local and regional providers. The medical community has come a long ways in the last 10 years for so many diseases and compromised health -care states. We are making much progress on many fronts but we still don't have all the answers.

There still can be breakthrough illnesses such as H1N1 and the Zika virus that can be transmitted from other species and pose a threat to anyone's health. By keeping your immune system strong, you reduce the risk of internally or externally generated conditions.

CHAPTER XI
SPIRITUALITY AND HEALING
"To find yourself, think for yourself" Socrates[13]

One of the things that I have come to believe over the past 4 1/2 years is the power of having faith for both spirituality and healing purposes. Persons of faith who are prayed for and who pray for themselves and others often seem to have better outcomes.

For most of us we know that prayers and spirituality are great expressions of faith, and help to keep you calm and also provide focus and direction to your healing and recovery efforts. I believe that prior to embarking on any type of serious recovery efforts from cancer or any debilitating disease, you should take a spiritual inventory first.

I affirm that having faith in God and believing in divine intervention has made my recovery efforts much more rooted. Through taking your personal inventory and embarking on a quest for spiritual recovery has to be the preface for the medical and physical portions of this recovery equation.

I also believe that it's conceivable to create a self-guided spirituality, but tapping other well established entities is like acquiring property on South Beach. It's well vetted already and just waiting for new tenants.

Finding that spiritual path paved the way for how I am now perceiving my illness. I no longer am so focused on "recovery". Although it would be great to have a full life again, whatever is in the cards is probably predetermined and just waiting for its fruition.

I now believe that daily "quiet" times with much spirituality on the menu and nightly prayers have been a positive daily staple in my life. I would be much more

---

[13] Socrates is a famous Greek philosopher

41

frustrated and confused about the future if I just relied on traditional medical model choices.

I pray to St. Francis, St. Peregrine, Father Mazzucchelli and others. I also go to the Sinsinawa Mound for prayer time and utilize their penance belt.

Each person can find what works for them, but I think it's a must that you know where you stand spiritually and are dedicated and sincere in your faith. For many of us, having a belief outside of yourself such as nature, the universe and painting can constitute "spirituality." But believing in God, from any denominational faith or religion will be a spiritual bonus for you.

Being loyal to your prayer rituals and having due diligence with this, will get easier and easier with time and practice. It is what it is and it's what you make of it that matters. You only can control your thoughts and actions, and I think that this is the most important investment that you will ever make.

How and why does a person get started with creating or enhancing his or her spiritual world? It's in your best interest at so many levels to have some spirituality in your life. I believe that your spiritual and healing worlds are linked (body, mind, spirit).

Spirituality in your life should be the focal point from where you pivot with important life decisions. It can be your safe zone where only spiritual strength and positive energy exists. Just listening to a sermon from an experienced preacher can inspire.

When you go from there, it's your "nirvana" with nothing toxic. When you have reached this place you can just let go of all earthly stressors and troubles. You can think of this as fuel for your healing system, because that's exactly what it is.

The healing system is abstractly viewed as an innate ability of your body's immune system, with its many tributaries to coalesce and bring to bear the many facets of itself that can restore your optima health. (Kind of like the Amazon River and its basin)

Remember that toxic emotional issues like anger, depression, and regret are all counterproductive to the healing ability. If you find yourself in the "flight or fight" mode, try not to stay there, because if this circumstance is activated often enough it will impede your healing efforts and cause even more distress. Even if you feel "justified" in your outrage, do what you can to return to the mindfulness or calm state, restoring homeostasis.

I would hope that it would be a moral imperative for anyone with a serious illness to have a sense of spirituality. A walk in the woods, painting, meditating all can be spiritual in nature. If you want to get your "mojo" back, you will have to embark on a spiritual healing journey along with medical and physical healing efforts.

Your memory muscle will be created and will pay dividends for you as you get more familiar and comfortable with use of some form of spirituality. I believe that we are all born with an innate sense of having an open mind to possibilities. We are creative without limits when in kindergarten and grade school.

It is later in adulthood when many of us get comfortable with our routines and lives when we reduce the spectrum of limitless possibilities. Going back in time and finding your place in the spiritual world can be a blessing for you.

Perhaps, a place to start is to get away from media influences and return to what has been fun for you as a child. Retapping your inquisitive nature can be a boon for this portion of your healing journey. The options are only limited to what restrictions that you place on them. Start now by "thinking outside of the box" and visualize yourself on a starship for the destination of the best you.

CHAPTER XII
GETTING REPURPOSED
"Man's Search for Meaning" Victor Frankl[14]

There will hopefully be a point on your journey in which you will be stabilized, keeping busy staying involved. Grabbing the handle on getting repurposed is an important fork in the road.

I want to congratulate anyone who has survived and is living with a chronic debilitating condition. Having suffered through the many ups and downs of your condition you may just think "Hey, I made it this far and I am just going to enjoy being alive."

Your jubilation is a normal part of your post -illness crisis and stabilization but there is more to be gained from having a meaningful and purposeful existence than just to say "I made it and am going to relax from now on".

I believe that most of us want to find opportunities to give back, be productive or at least be useful to our families and society. You probably can't return to your prior job and may face many limitations, but there are more "cans" than "cannots".

You can no longer run, but you can walk; you can no longer play basketball but you can water walk. Keeping active and finding fun, creative ways to stay in the game is as important as any medication you are taking or any therapy you would be getting.

Finding my way after being so active and involved has been a character building experience. Working through painful experiences and accepting new limitations was difficult for me. There were a lot of moments of doubt and

---

[14] Victor Frankl was a POW survivor and psychiatrist

frustration. Accepting the "new normal" and working within those parameters has gotten easier with time.

Growing up in the 1960's in Iowa for me and many of us was like going to a living history farm. From JFK'S assassination of 1963 to Dr. King's and Bobby Kennedy's deaths in 1968 and the moon landing, life was full of cultural and social events. Some of these were enriching and some were tragic.

The vocational and educational "norms" expressed during that time period were to complete your education, get a good job, have a family and career and retire for the good life. It was just not scripted to have a life altering disease and be off of the playing field.

I have found that a combination of exercise, spirituality, family, social and friendship involvements has helped me to feel good about who I am at this age and stage of my recovery. There may be a point in time, in which I might need hospice or palliative care. So when there comes a time for a "life review" I think it would be good to be able to reflect on every age, milestone, setback and opportunity to believe that I did my best with the cards I was dealt.

There also will likely be times when others who have or are a caregiver for a person with a debilitating condition may experience compassion fatigue. I did experience a sense of physical and psychological tiredness on many occasions.

The long months between appointments, bone and CT scans can be filled with worry and stress. A person may want to give up or just get so tired with waiting and hoping for healing that they just experience a numbness. This emotion can be part of the grief and loss process or may occur at various stages during your protracted treatment.

I have found it useful to look back and reflect on getting this far and to have gratitude for being alive. I also am diligent at taking "one day at a time" and just doing what I can for now and believing that tomorrow will take care of itself.

It's probably more difficult to watch a loved one waste away with a debilitating condition, such as Alzheimer's. Both of my parents died with forms of dementia and during their final years it truly was wrenching to see them slowly decompensate. Watching your loved ones lose physical and mental abilities can definitely drain a caregiver's energy and vitality.

Compassion fatigue indicates a form of "burn out" but not in the work related sense, instead the emotional and physical caregiving sense. When you visit your loved ones and they hardly recognize you and are struggling with basic activities of daily living it could be contributing to this type of fatigue.

Over a period of time being a primary caregiver and perhaps doing collateral things like paying the bills, mowing the lawn and shoveling the snow can wear a person out. Another term that is used at times is the "sandwich generation". This would mean taking care of kids and parents at the same time.

Whatever the term that is being used and whether it's experienced with your own condition or the condition of a loved one, the impact will affect the same psychological and emotional domains. This reaction is completely normal and it's very important to recognize that if it is happening to you it's not a sign of weakness. There should be no shame in taking an inventory of what you are doing for whom and what you are experiencing.

The next step would be to redistribute the emotional and physical workloads to family, neighbors, friends or professionals. There are a variety of agencies that can coordinate caregivers or help steer the son or daughter in the direction of community resources and support options. Be sure to take time for self-care on a regular basis.

If you the caregiver who also has a long-term debilitating illness you might realize that you have been afflicted with compassion fatigue. You may then need to give yourself permission to take corrective action.

I always felt that I should be the caregiver and provider to others in my family who have needed the help, especially during the last several years. I have a disabled brother who lives in a group home, with whom I am co-guardian for. Although this is a labor of love, it's also stressful to get phone calls of his deteriorating condition.

Also during the last several years I was one of the primary caregivers for my mother, who lived on her own until age 88 and was always very independent. It was a struggle for her to accept limits in her life, like not being able to drive, or play cards or live independently anymore.

In my healing journey, I have learned to pace myself, ask others for help, give myself permission for more "self-care" and just try to distribute what time and energy is available in the most productive ways possible. There may never be a sense of completion or perfection in these endeavors, but knowing that you have helped to ease others, suffering or loneliness, can be emotionally and psychologically restorative.

There are no guarantees in the future if you follow what you consider the optimal healing and wellness course. If you do everything that I have listed in this book and other things that you find useful, there is still uncontrollable events.

Believing that every day is precious and every relationship and interaction is important may serve you like it has me in my healing journey. Making today count and living life to the fullest with no regrets and no resentments certainly makes sense.

I have come to the point of radical self -acceptance and am seeking to find fulfillment and growth opportunities when they present themselves. Writing this book was partly inspired by a close friend who told me of his journey with relationships, emotions and frustrations.

I do believe that journaling and prayer are just two of many useful tools that a person can cultivate over time. Each of us will have to find what works from a lot of choices. It was important for me to not get stuck at a certain stage or process of recovering from cancer. Even though I still have stage 4 cancer, I believe that I have coped as well as can be expected. If things get terminal for me from a cancer perspective, I just pray to God that I can finish this journey with as much dignity and grace as the creator has bestowed upon me.